A Lullaby

Praeclarus Press, LLC
2504 Sweetgum Lane
Amarillo, Texas 79124 USA
806-367-9950
www.PraeclarusPress.com

DISCLAIMER

The information contained in this publication is advisory only and is not intended to replace sound clinical judgment or individualized patient care. The author disclaims all warranties, whether expressed or implied, including any warranty as the quality, accuracy, safety, or suitability of this information for any particular purpose.

ISBN: 978-1-946665-51-5

Cover Design: Ken Tackett
Developmental Editing: Kathleen Kendall-Tackett
Copyediting: Chris Tackett
Layout & Design: Nelly Murariu

A Lullaby

Reflections for Caregivers of Breastfeeding Families

Chris Auer

Praeclarus Press, LLC

www.PraeclarusPress.com

Under one sky
there's a baby's cry,
under one sky,
a mother's lullaby,
under one sky
we are all a part of everything.

- Musical Excerpt:
Under One Sky by Chris Barton

The first line on the previous page is the title of my first book. Using nature as a perspective, it conveys that everything and everyone belongs. We are more the same than different. That's not to diminish what makes us unique, such as our DNA, temperament, family history, culture, or story. But doesn't this moment in life, in place and in time, continue to compel us to seek unity?

Through our work with moms and babies, we have been given a wide-angled lens to see more clearly where our commonalities converge. The book you hold invites you to spend some time reflecting on the small picture: What this period of your journey supporting breast-pumping and breastfeeding families means, *and* what *you* might need. It also encourages you to reflect on the big picture – union. The baby is united with the mom in the womb, in the latch, and in babywearing. Mothers are united with other mothers by fundamental common hopes and experiences. Families are united to families by the thread of desire for a happy, loving, safe, and meaningful life. We, as well, are united in our commitment to families.

In *Under One Sky*, the epigraphs were used as springboards to tell the story of mothers from many countries and walks of life. The purpose of this book is to reflect on *our* story as lactation consultants, peers, midwives, physicians, researchers, nutritionists, La Leche League leaders, nurses, physical/occupational therapists, lactation counselors, and simply, human beings. We, who assist and nurture from the early hours of this new bond to the weaning stage, transmit more than information and technique. In these relatively brief encounters, we transmit values that a mother can carry well beyond breastfeeding. We often have opportunities to demonstrate patience, acceptance, appreciation, surrender, gratitude, respect, perseverance, attentiveness, and so on. We provide important care. Trust that. Trust yourself.

Our encounters with breastfeeding families are also teaching us new understandings of the complexity of our work. Yet, if we are attentive, they are awakening us to connect with our own soul work.

When do we need to take a breath, find courage and hope, ask for supervision, seek honest feedback, get some space, be receptive to new ideas, listen better, or listen to our own heart's desire?

This book offers you an opportunity for reflection and self-care. Each week holds two reflections. I hope it can be a vehicle for you to center yourself before diving into the day. In fact, I hope it pulls you back a bit from operating from a rushed space. Some days, we are in a blessed and good space. Some days, we are in a difficult personal space that we cannot see until retrospect, where the hidden gift might lie. Still, we go about our work. Some evenings, we collapse into bed with sweet dreams ahead. Some evenings, we find ourselves doing a mental recap of the day. I hope this book encourages those moments. Your examination of your day's work shouldn't be a pass/ fail test. It can be a way of noticing moments that brought you an insight, a moment of awe or nudge that your ship's rudder may need to be altered for you to stay headed toward your True North.

If you're a morning person, then as the songbirds are singing, may reading a reflection invite you to step back, pause, and consider what your inner wisdom is saying. If you're a night owl, I hope that this book can be an evening's lullaby, helping you to draw perspective and inspiration. In either case, inserting a reflective pause is a worthy act of love that may begin with you but extends itself into our world.

—Chris Auer, March, 2021

christineauer952@gmail.com

ACKNOWLEDGMENTS

Thank you to my colleagues who didn't just complete their required continuing education but grew as people through their self-reflection and sharing of their stories. To borrow from Carl Jung, "Who looks inside, awakes."

Thank you to Praeclarus Press for believing enough in the value of reflection to take on this project.

Thank you to Ken Tackett for the art illustrations in this book.

Thank you to Susan Mueller for her editorial insights and for saving me from my pronoun-challenged self.

Thank you to all the mothers, fathers, and babies who taught me to be in the *now* and gave me a reason to reflect on our encounters.

Thank you to my adult children—Jen, Amy, Andrew, and Jason, as well as Nicole—who help me be a better person and inspire me to live my values.

Thank you to my grandchildren—Ava, Nate, Abby, and Olivia—who enrich my life beyond measure.

Thank you to Ron, who patiently waits for me to come back to the *now* of our life together.

Dedication

With gratitude to Richard Rohr,
Franciscan mentor, and friend, for 50 years
of helping me appreciate the sacred and
teachable moments in all encounters
if I but pause, look, and listen.

CONTENTS

CONTENTS

Gratitude

I'm embarrassed to be doing so much beautiful work.
Seldom has a human being been so fortunate.

- Albert Schweitzer

We are fortunate, indeed. Remember that when you are weary. Think about the last amazing interaction with a family. Who gets this much gratification? Isn't it so true that we receive at least as much as we give? Even on nights when you lie in bed thinking of things you could have done better, you were there, giving your all. Celebrate that with a good night's sleep tonight.

We persist and live longer than we think, leaving traces
of ourselves wherever we go.

- Dinaw Mengestu, *How to Read the Air*

There will be times when a multipara mom remembers you, but right now, spend a moment considering who influenced *you* to be the professional you are today. Who has left a footprint on your career path? Who inspired you to make a commitment to human lactation? Close your eyes. Picture them. What did they say or model that empowered you? Breathe out a thank you. And if you're lucky enough to still be in touch with them, consider dropping them a line. Begin your day with gratitude.

Hope

Sometimes in the middle of nothing, hope breaks through and gives you something.

- Ethiopian woman, *Oxfam Homepage*

Hope doesn't always spring eternal. Some days can be trying. Look for places of hope even while there is background noise in parts of society being critical of breastfeeding, which is truly sad. Feel it, but don't dwell there. Your ability to be present is highly influenced by where you allow your mind to focus. May hope break through for you the next time that things look dark. You are not alone, either. Remember, there is an *international community that believes in your work. We believe in you.*

This world is full of conflicts and full of things that cannot be reconciled. But there are moments when we can . . . reconcile and embrace the whole mess . . . and that's what I call Hallelujah.

- Leonard Cohen

If you are in the lactation field, you are likely familiar with the 3 Ps: policy, protocol, and procedure. While they are meant to create continuity, certitude, and clarity, they are nothing without accountability. If you have good ones, consider yourself lucky. If you work somewhere with antiquated policies, then you are probably working as a change agent while embracing the "whole mess." Otherwise, you'll become disgruntled, disillusioned, and distraught. Your time is better spent. Like other fields, the lactation world has its share of frustrations and contradictions from within, including our professional organizations and the logistics of reimbursement and recertification. We can't fix it all, and certainly, we can't fix it all at once. Breathe.

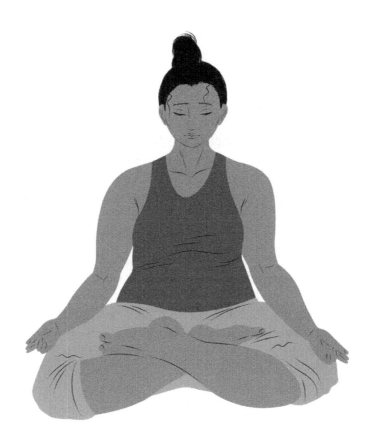

Touch

I've learned that every day, you should reach out and touch someone.

- Maya Angelou

... with permission, of course! But let's start back when your day is just beginning. Who is your very first contact? A partner, a pet, a child, the person in your complex's parking lot leaving for work the same time as you, or the stranger in the employee parking garage? I'm guessing that it's not your client/patient/couplet. There are so many opportunities to touch someone. I'm not a morning person. In fact, on the drive to my high school, my father would often ask my sister, "What's with grumpy over there?" (This many years past, still something I'm not proud of.) We each have to find our way to the sweet spot where we can touch and be touched daily.

The lactation field is full of people with open hearts. How you create receptivity each day is a sacred underpinning of your work. But I also hope you find ways to keep the heart space open at the dawn of your day so you can reach out and touch those in your inner circle, be that family, a pet, a neighbor, or a colleague.

Culture is the blueprint for human behavior.

- Jan Riordan

Why are metaphors so effective in communication? "He's as punctual as a Swiss watch. She's as manicured as a Japanese garden. They exude the *joie de vivre* of every Parisian." These immediately create *context* and images, which then help us interpret what we are seeing. This can help us immensely in a given lactation consult. Understanding a mother's cultural context goes beyond the country. Still, it begins with understanding her national heritage. Remembering that a Latina mother will not want ice water after the birth, you offer her warm teas or natural drinks. But this doesn't help you understand why a woman of a similar background to you isn't following your feeding plan. I've asked many a grandma and *father*, "What do you think Mom and baby need right now?" Who's influencing the mother? They may not even be present. It could be a voice in her head. Lots of cultural frameworks are unconscious and ingrained. Helping a mother uncover the values that drive her decisions is a gift we can give her as she navigates the uncharted waters of parenting and breastfeeding. It's also a reminder to examine what and who shapes our decisions.

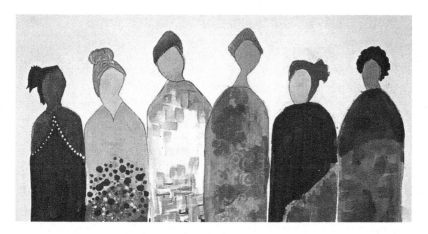

Fear

Some people feel the rain; others just get wet.

- Bob Marley

There is prudent caution, and then there is fear. What's holding you back? Of course, this is a question that could go well beyond your career. Here are some common roadblocks to *feeling the rain*.

"I am afraid I won't be successful."

"I worry about other people's opinions of me."

"I need to play it safe."

"It takes too much energy."

"What if I'm not as needed as before?"

"What if it affects my livelihood?"

"What if I'm wrong?"

There's another question you might ask yourself.

"What will bring me the most joy?"

Loving and accepting who you are in the moment doesn't preclude challenging yourself to make a leap of faith if a leap of faith is called for. Just don't forget to have an umbrella handy if you start experiencing a deluge before you see the rainbow!

*Believing that baby formula is as good as breast milk is
believing that 30 years of technology is superior to
3 million years of nature's evolution.*

- Christina Northrup

I suppose I'd have to modify this now by saying it's been 90 years, but that's a drop in the bucket compared to 3 *million* years. There are things to be grateful for; formula is no longer made with Karo syrup and evaporated milk. We know that we shouldn't introduce cow's milk before age one. There have been advancements in 90 years. Formula isn't bad; breast milk is simply superior. Unfortunately, we compete with a 90-billion-dollar industry that finds insidious ways to market to mothers. I heard a physician from South Africa speak recently who said that they had to make a country-wide ban on formula gifts to stem infant deaths.

We all agree we don't want mothers whose babies need a supplement to be afraid to provide it. On the flip side, we don't want mothers to be afraid to breastfeed exclusively. Each year, we learn more about the intricate components of human milk, from immunoglobulins to T-cells to oligosaccharides. Every journal article and well-designed study further affirms our efforts are worth it. Your efforts are worth it. Her efforts are worth it.

Compassion

The future is sending back good wishes and waiting with open arms.

- Kobi Yamada

Reread this epigraph. Take it in. Let it empower you to forge ahead in your mission, your research, your publishing, and your one-to-one mother-baby encounters. Some days are 3 steps forward and 1 step back, but the universe is headed in the direction of the common good, and being in this field, we are a part of that forward momentum.

You say gently to yourself: This person has feelings, emotions, and thoughts – just like me. This person at some point in his or her life, has been sad, disappointed, hurt or confused – just like me. This person has, in his or her life, experienced physical and emotional pain and suffering – just like me.

- Chade-Menge Tan

This quote from a *Google* engineer speaks to me about compassion, receptivity, and teamwork. If it reminds you of mothers you serve who are on the edges of society, it applies even more.

But consider administrators, supervisors, and managers who were not *all in* on breastfeeding. Sometimes you aren't in a position to influence decisions that, once made, have an unintended negative effect on breastfeeding dyads. I have tried to take a breath and not be overly reactive, with varying degrees of success. I try to remember that they are juggling many competing values: operational efficiency, budget, and limited staffing while still trying to uphold the organization's mission statement. Their lens is different than ours. We can react, or we can step back and figure out how to work collaboratively. This is the Quadrant 1 work that Stephen Covey speaks of: Addressing the Important but Not Urgent. It is painstaking, and we don't always see decision reversals. It's well worth our time to build a broad base of stakeholders so we aren't swimming upstream alone. Our lens is breastfeeding success, exclusivity, and best practice. We can meet our managers on the playing field of Best Practice.

Done Enough

I have done what is mine to do.

- Saint Francis of Assisi

I remember seeing the movie *Schindler's List* and watching in awe at a depth of regret portrayed by Schindler when the war was over, feeling that he *could have done more* to save more Jews in his country. These were extreme circumstances, yet on a much tinier scale, haven't you gotten to the end of your day and thought, "I could have done more?" It takes a bit of humility to say that you did the best you could today. We have twinges of doubt that all will be well when we return the next day. These are often credible concerns. Yet, we have to put the mother into the loving care of her instincts, as well as to those who will be around her, and to know that tomorrow, we'll roll up our sleeves for whatever her situation needs at the moment.

Still, there is the next generation of lactation providers to consider. Francis followed this statement made to his brothers at the end of his life by saying that now they, in turn, must do what it is theirs to do. We know it's important to do our part to prepare those who will come after us. Like the mothers and babies that we leave at the end of a shift, we want to walk away, knowing that we have done what was ours to do. That's a grace worth asking for.

Have a big enough heart to love unconditionally, and a broad enough mind to embrace the differences that make us unique.

- D. B. Harrop

Do you notice that your practice is similar to some practitioners and remarkably different than others? How do you respond? The field of lactation, like medicine, is a combination of science and art. It's the art side that makes us approach consults with a different twist. Is one wrong and the other right? Most often not, but it's hard to overcome the bias of the way I do things or even the bias of "the way we've always done it here." Some LCs' strength is in bedside teaching. Some have strengths to engage the extended family in meaningful ways. Some have strengths to negotiate for change with management. We can't wear all hats. The trick is to identify who has what strengths, back away with an open mind, and allow them their moment to steer the boat.

Listening

I'd like it to be thought that I listened carefully to what patients and others have told me, that I've tried to imagine what it was like for them, and that I tried to convey this.

- Doctor Oliver Sachs

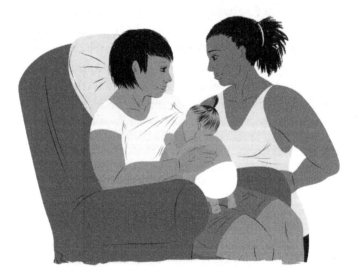

If someone isn't listening to you on this level, you risk running on empty. So first, consider seeking out that someone who will be a listening presence for you. It's healing. Remember the adage, "Physician, heal thyself?" Start here. Let peace begin with you. You're worth it.

Extending this model of empathic listening takes time to cultivate. Our brain chatter can easily get in the way. After all, we've heard countless similar stories but not the one from this particular mom. Our belief that we have the answer before the mom even finishes sharing gets in the way too. I have often referred to a silly YouTube video called *It's Not About the Nail*, to bring home this point. It's effective. Check it out! It reminds us that we must resist jumping in to fix and problem solve until we've addressed her most fundamental need: to be heard.

Remember me as the one who woke up.

- Buddha

It is hugely rewarding when we've been the conduit of an ah-ha moment. A mom now understands how unnecessary supplements can create the downward spiral of the very thing she fears: not having enough. Or she realizes that picking her baby up when he's crying won't make him dependent, code for "spoiling" him. Rather, picking him up makes him feel safe and helps him grow toward independence in its proper time. "Wake up!" we would like to say; babies are inherently dependent.

Don't we, too, have our ah-ha moments? Close your eyes a moment and consider your last one. Has this helped you as a practitioner, parent, partner, employee, boss, or human being? What a gift, right?

Acceptance

Knowing that we can be loved exactly as we are gives us all the best opportunity for growing into the healthiest of people.

- Fred Rogers

Consider the baby in your care. Acceptance begins here. Modeling that begins with us. Example: "No, your baby isn't lazy. He's just sleepy." Asking a mom what her heart is telling her often helps her find her inner wisdom—helping a mom understand that there are phases in infancy that pass can give her an anchor to hang onto during sleep-deprived nights. It's not the baby's fault. It just is. Loving this tiny creature entrusted to us also means loving the Now, whatever that is.

Now consider the mom. Maybe she is someone who has an unidentified cause for her low supply. She feels terrible, like she's not a good enough mom. You work with her using every tool in your toolbox. It doesn't change. Helping her surrender to what is may become the most important intervention you offer her. Her worth is intrinsic. It isn't based on the volume of her milk or the success of a latch. It just is. Show her. Tell her.

What do you pack to pursue a dream and what do you leave behind?

- Sandra Sharpe

There's always a trade-off, isn't there? Evenings we spend reading some of the latest research or studying for an exam is in place of something else in your life. You may have 5 values consistent with another LC or with your partner, but if you prioritize them differently, your journey will look quite different than that of the person next to you. Try not to leave people behind. Try to appreciate what they value. That will go a long way in understanding behavior. Think about your top 5 values. What's the dream that's driving you? Consider the values reflected by someone you respect. What's the dream that's driving them?

Culture

A nation's culture lies in the hearts and the souls of its people.

- Mahatma Gandhi

So, how would you describe your country's culture? What makes a whole swath of folks generous, kindhearted, responsible, or playful? But also, consider the population you serve. Is it diverse or homogenous? What (or who) makes their hearts beat? Another way to consider this is to reflect on what brings out the best in people? When you answer that personally, you may be getting at a part of yourself that has absorbed the culture of your own nation. How does that serve you in your lactation work? Does it make you more compassionate or compulsively prompt? Has it given you that third eye that can sense there's more to the story than what a mother is offering up? Is there any way that it's a hindrance, such as inclining you to be judgmental of those who think or do things differently than you? We can all agree that one thing that makes each mother's heartbeat is her children. Here's one place we all meet.

There are a hundred different ways to kneel and kiss the ground.

- Rumi

In *Under One Sky*, I did not include the sentence prior to the one above: *let the beauty we love be what we do*. I have no doubt that those who serve breastfeeding families have a passion for what they do. We each express it differently, whether that be through volunteer work in mom groups such as *Baby Café*, in outpatient hospital settings, maternity wards, research, mentoring, home visits, dental offices, milk banks, or conference planning. The list is nearly endless. It takes a village of us. Honor our diversity: setting, style, ethnicity, and gender.

Mothers also teach us to honor the diverse ways they approach and hopefully meet their breastfeeding goals. The goals themselves are diverse and sometimes not ones we'd choose for a mom, but it is *her* journey to find her unique way to kneel and kiss the ground.

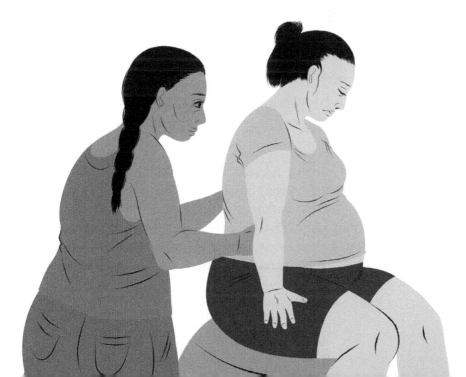

Stories

I am the interpreter of stories. - Nat King Cole

What sleuths we are in the world of lactation! At times, trying to piece the puzzle together to identify the root cause is confounding. Be sure to celebrate your ah-ha moments when one sidebar of information a mom provides suddenly sheds light so that you can see the puzzle in its entirety. I find it especially interesting to hear about a mom's past experience with breastfeeding. Is she interpreting her current situation based on the past? Can she create a self-fulfilling prophecy? Or is it raising red flags for you too? What then? It's tricky to know how much optimism to express when you can't guarantee an outcome. Still, I think that hope should be our compass. Hope in the grander scheme that *all will be well.*

If you can dream it, you can do it. - Walt Disney

The first step to realizing a dream is to visualize that it's achievable. Trust yourself. Believe in your mission, but don't hesitate to expand that mission or to pay attention to that different dream creeping into the corner of your mind. It can be both scary and invigorating to pivot and take a hard look at a new urging. Believe that the places you're called to realize a dream are the places where you feel a profound gladness.

Connecting

When life descends into the pit, I must be my own candle,
willingly burning myself to light up the darkness around me.

- Alice Walker

As I write, we are now in week 4 of a state lockdown due to the global pandemic. Our governor has just challenged us to contact 5 people each day who may need connection. I've just launched a virtual lactation consulting service that is gratis. Even before the launch, I'd had communiques from two women who'd delivered the same day, ten days prior: one in Cincinnati, one outside of Ohio. One was a primipara, and the other had a 2-year-old. It's lonely out there for new moms, and it definitely can feel like the pit when you are having breastfeeding issues and traditional services are shut down. I know not everyone is in a position to offer complementary services, but many of us know moms whom we've helped who would benefit from a call. In the scheme of things, the balance between you reaching out or waiting for a mom to initiate may tip in favor of you being first to reach out. You may be that candle lighting the way.

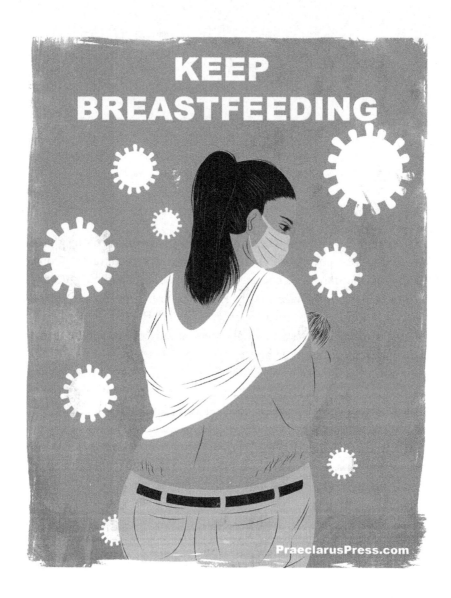

If the only prayer you ever said in your life was, "Thank You," that would be enough.

- Meister Eckhart

Begin each day with gratitude. Here's my litany; "thank you for my health and wellbeing. Thank you for the sun creeping through the clouds and the weather warming. Thank you to all those who work on the frontlines for breastfeeding families. Thank you to the colleagues in other fields who share this work. Thank you for a career that's not just a job but a passion. Thank you to the mothers who place their trust in us. Thank you to the colleagues who work behind the scene in research, our professional organizations, the WHO, the scientists, and the authors who publish new findings. Thank you to those who support me on my own home front: family, friends, and spiritual companions. Thank you for my other interests that keep me sane and grounded."

What would you add?

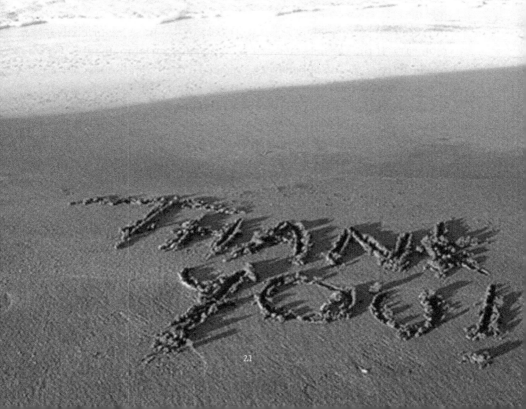

Teachable Moments

A pair of substantial mammary glands has the advantage over the two hemispheres of the most learned professor's brain in the art of compounding a nutritive fluid for infants.

- Oliver Wendell Holmes

By the way, they don't have to be "substantial." I'm not fond of simplified arguments over the content of human milk versus artificial milk. For example, there is less iron in mothers' milk. A medical student told me this. He seemed to think it was a "gotcha moment," not taking into account bioavailability. Try your best to see these as teachable moments. If they aren't, they can become adversarial moments. We need partners. We need believers. We need a coalition. It does take a village. Tread with care in these situations. Artificial milk has its place. We don't need to be convinced of that. If only we had the marketing money that the corporations have. Wouldn't that be something? What would your human milk slogan be?

Life is a tapestry we weave day by day with threads of different colors, some heavy and dark, others thin and bright, all threads having their uses. The stupid things I did are already in the tapestry, indelible, but I'm not going to be weighed down by them til I die. What's done is done. I have to look ahead.

-Isabel Allende

You are human. You make mistakes. Forgive yourself. If necessary, apologize. Learn the lesson to be learned and move on. We all wish for do-overs. They generally don't happen. But, sometimes, life surprises us by putting us in similar situations and inviting a different response. So, yes, I think we can add some bright colors to the tapestry of our lives by choosing different responses, different actions, and thus, different outcomes. Sometimes we have to just be humble enough to admit the stupidity.

Seeing Beneath

A poor widow came in and put in two small copper coins which amounted to a cent . . . out of her poverty she put in all that she owned.

- Jesus Christ

To borrow from another parable, what is the pearl of great price for you? What will you pay to own it? This is a question for you alone to answer. When have you been that widow putting in all that you have with only faith that it will be worth it?

You may have known mothers whose pearl itself is breastfeeding. Blest are you who companion someone on one such journey. It can be both inspiring and heartbreaking to witness the struggle as she puts in all that she has.

I am done with great things and big things with great institutions and big success. And I am for those tiny, invisible, molecular moral forces that work from individual to individual through the crannies of the world.

- William James

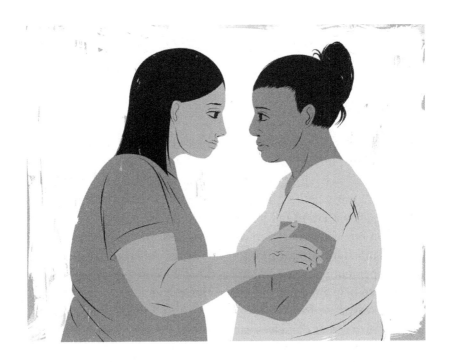

You may work for one of those "great institutions." All well and good, but grace begins locally, one interaction at a time. When you offer a listening presence, while it may be invisible, it is the crack that allows the light to enter. Being in emotional proximity is a gift, even beyond the latch and corrected positioning. To stay with the mom in the moment sometimes opens us to another way of seeing what is happening underneath, giving way to an inspired recommendation, a new insight, or a new sense of compassion.

Inner Peace

My husband is a pivotal anchor in my life. His influence encourages me to be independent and take risks.

- Padmasree Warrior

I originally used this quote to be juxtaposed to a dad who, being vehemently against breastfeeding, walked out when I was demonstrating position and latch with the mom-baby couplet. The significant others in a mom's life, whether the father, partner, or grandma, are pivotal anchors. They seem to fall into three categories: supportive, neutral (based on no prior experience with breastfeeding), or overtly critical. As with this dad, we can gently try to explore their reasons and correct misperceptions, but we can't control the outcome. Pregnancy is the time to help a mom develop her network of support and create a strategic response to naysayers. That's being proactive. Spending a little time to center ourselves each day gives us a better chance to be responsive and not reactive to critics.

Serenity Now!- George Costanza, *Seinfeld*

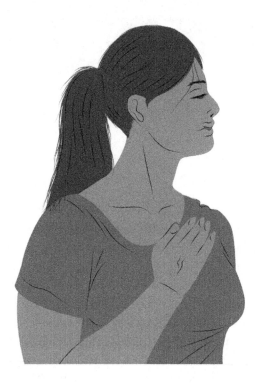

I keep a cartoon image in my phone's photo gallery. It's a woman in the lotus pose, meditating. It reads, "C'mon inner peace. I haven't got all day!" Isn't that usually the way it is? Frustrating moments that trigger a negative response in us happen so abruptly. Instead of opting to reply with equal spontaneity, here's an idea; insert a pause. Take a breath and another. If your life includes small children, it may not be reasonable to meditate. Consider beginning by just taking one conscious breath each morning. It'll go a long way.

Unknowing

Being at ease with not knowing is crucial for answers to come to you.

- Eckart Tolle

A friend of mine first saw Mr. Tolle on an Oprah Winfrey series. After that, he affectionately referred to him as "the guy in the Mr. Rogers sweater." Seriously, as the author of *The Power of Now*, he reminds us that *now* is all we have. When we adopt an attitude of unknowing, we listen to a mom without preconceived ideas of the solution to her problem. We hone in. We listen with all our senses, not just our ears. We allow wisdom, hers and ours, to slip in through the silence of a pregnant pause. Practice it today with someone – family, colleague, or parent. In the end, though, we still have to be okay with mystery.

A hero is simply someone who rises above his or her own human weaknesses, for an hour, a day, a year, to do something stirring.

- Betty Deramus

Give praise to the heroes. Don't we learn that in any crisis? Think about your workplace. Who's a hero there? Sometimes it's obvious. Still, don't forget to notice the people who, working in unexpected places, go above and beyond the call of duty to support breastfeeding.

I once gave an "Ask Me About Breastfeeding" lapel button to one of our environmental staff because she was so sweet to let me know about moms she thought needed to be seen sooner than later. How did she know this? By being a good listener. As she mopped floors, she became attuned to cues that a mom was wavering or had an unsupportive significant other, or some shared concerns about their sore nipples. She had no personal experience with breastfeeding, but she didn't allow how she fed her own babies to influence her commitment to care for these women.

Addiction

No one is immune from addiction: it afflicts people of all ages, races, classes, professions.

— Patrick Kennedy

Most of us in the U. S. have spent time sheltering in place, per orders from our governors and health advisors. I can't help but read this quote in that light. Anyone else find that too much time at home leads to looking aimlessly into the food pantry? Of course, Patrick Kennedy is referring to drug and alcohol recovery. Many of us have helped women in recovery as they breastfeed or pump for their newborns. They have both unique needs and the same needs as any other mom. If you serve this particular demographic of women, you are not alone. The struggle of recovery is everywhere, and unfortunately, the medical community, with its overprescribing of opiates, bears some of the responsibility. It's easy to slip into judgment unless you can widen your heart to find your common humanity with these moms.

Before you can break out of prison, you must first realize you are locked up.

— Unknown

Addiction takes many forms, including being addicted to my way of thinking. Over time, we learn that there is more than one way to conduct a lactation consult (or a life). There is more than one way to design a good human milk study, at least sometimes. One of the gifts of mentoring new LCs is to see the plethora of ways we relate to mothers. What newbie has taught you something you didn't know or give you a style to admire? That's a gift, and it saddens me when I hear interns say that they don't feel taken seriously because they're new in the profession. Let's not "eat our young." After all, we're counting on them to bear the torch we will one day pass on to them.

What is it that you might detach from to be a healthier you?

Insecurity

I am convinced that virtually every destructive behavior and addiction I battled off and on for years was rooted in my insecurity.

- Beth Moore

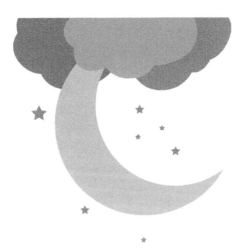

This epigraph precedes another breastfeeding and addiction story from *Under One Sky*. As I considered this, it occurred to me that part of our commonality is that we each occasionally chose behaviors or reactions that don't serve our true selves. It may be a slight or a hurtful comment of a colleague or an adult child. However unintentional, we notice a tug, or maybe even a small adrenalin surge, as we consider saying something we'll regret later. I've included the word "lullaby" in this book's title because many of us don't have time for a short reflection until the day's end. As you look back on the day, how can you reframe that event so it will tap into your most secure and highest self? We all have our wounds, don't we?

Life is what happens when your cell phone is charging.

- Unknown

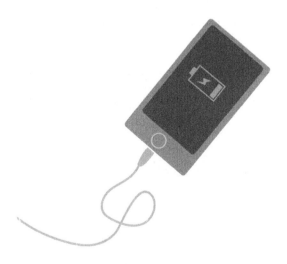

It's difficult to be present to the moment when we are preoccupied with the dings on that dang phone. We all agree; it's not black and white. When we use the phone to stay connected to real people in real-time, and not their online presence, it's a beautiful thing. If we use it for lactation purposes, who would fault that? But when does it interfere? When is it a distraction from who is right in front of you? When are you attending to social media instead of [you fill in the blank]? The scenario hardest to watch is a parent ignoring their child because the phone has ensnared them. It takes discipline to put boundaries on technology—something to think about in our quiet downtime moments.

Passion

People who never get carried away, should be!

- Malcomb Forbes

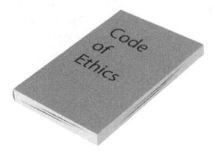

Remember when lactation was your first love? When you talked to a mom and suddenly more time than you had to give had been given anyway? Did you not walk away rejuvenated (and buzzing to get on to your next responsibility)? We are passionate about mother-baby health. There's the umbrella. It's disheartening to be called a breastfeeding zealot, or worse. Don't let other people's labels steal your passion. It's a gift. I trust that your enthusiasm doesn't blind you to the nutritional needs of any baby. I trust that you let science inform your recommendations. Trust your commitment to our Code of Ethics and Scope of Practice.

Crying would be pointless if mothers weren't genetically programmed to respond to it . . . the mother, the father, even strangers feel moved when a baby cries.

- Dr. Carlos Gonzalez, *Kiss Me*

Sometimes the most important advice you can give a mother is to listen to her heart. When outside voices are telling her to let him cry it out, you may be the only counterpoint. Then again, in the early days when she is nursing up a storm, and he's inconsolable, she's relying on you to understand her risk factors for low supply and sort out what is going on, or refer her back to the baby's care provider. You are both the lactation clinician and the midwife, helping to birth this new mom.

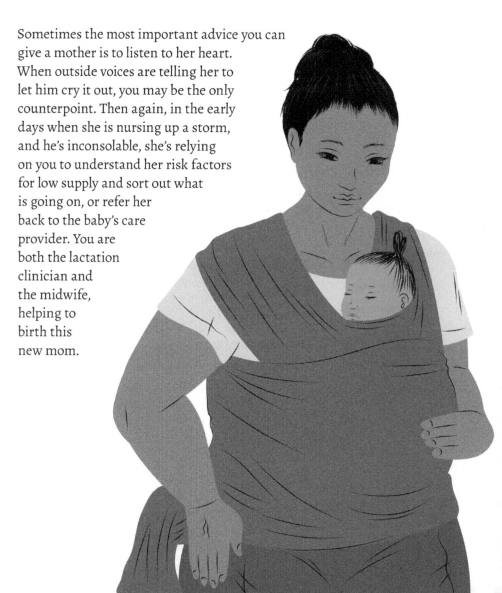

Reframing

By perseverance the snail reached the ark.

- Charles Spurgeon

What do you bemoan for taking so long? Where is it hard to see progress? Pace yourself.

On the mom's side, I knew a mother whose own mother was an excellent newborn intensive care nurse who breastfed eight children. This mom had a preemie with a 3-week NICU stay. Neither the mom nor the experienced grandma could get that baby to latch. Mom pumped religiously. When the baby was 3 months old, she picked her up while still undressed after showering. It was an unplanned gesture simply to answer the phone. As she spoke to the caller, her baby latched with no fuss whatsoever. Yeah!

We both know it doesn't always go this way. You can make a big difference by reframing what the "ark" is. It might be breastfeeding, chest-feeding, having enough milk, or it might be coming to a peace that whatever the moment holds, it's as perfect as it can be. She's counting on your wisdom.

Breastfeeding is a natural safety net against poverty . . .
It's almost as if breastfeeding takes the infant out of
poverty for those first few months in order to give the
child a fairer start in life to compensate for the injustice
of the world into which it was born.

- James Grant, past-President of UNICEF

Think about this. A milk bank would never be able to quantify the difference between milk from a poor or affluence donor mom. Mothers around the world have an equal chance of establishing breastfeeding. In fact, on this point alone, being in a developing country has notable advantages. What's more, isn't it amazing to witness the joy and sense of accomplishment when any mom, but particularly a first-time low-income mom, latches her baby successfully? It may be one of her first experiences of empowerment. How gratifying to witness!

Empowering

Assume the best, find common ground and find human connection. If we can find that grace, anything is possible.

- Barack Obama

In her 2019 research article, "The Alchemy of Connection," Indira Lopez-Bassols, reminds us that language is the foundation of the bridge and interaction between the LC and the mother. By being fully present and listening with an open mind, we perceive not just the "thread of the chief complaint" but also subtler cues that lead to further emotional and psychological concerns, thus developing a broader understanding and interpretation of the situations she presents. Connecting empowers a mother to take an active role in developing her breastfeeding care plan. The irony is that by connecting, we actually promote self-efficacy and independence.

Everyone has to make their own decisions. I still believe in that.

- Grace Jones

Have you ever felt a mom to be on the verge of successful breastfeeding when she quite unexpectedly decides to quit? Boy, that can be so disappointing when you feel like she's "almost there." Everyone has their tipping point when trying to achieve something. Sometimes they're less dramatic. Then there are our own life decisions. A sense of responsibility can cloud the need to take a step back. Do you have a decision looming in the background of your life right now? It takes courage to follow your gut when it's leading you to uncharted territory. Is it time to put your ear down next to your soul?

Praise

In the midst of winter, I found there was within me an invincible summer.

- Albert Camus

Praise for the mothers who demonstrate immeasurable fortitude. Praise for persistence and patience. Praise for the micro-preemies who have likely fought the most difficult battle of their lives. Praise for the mothers who exclusively pump, whether that be for their preemie, due to return to work or not achieving a latch, or simply, preference. Praise for the lactation support you provide those mothers who need to get through their "winters." Praise for the fathers or partners who are encouraging when the going is tough. Praise for healthcare providers who protect breastfeeding. Praise for the lactation network who pick up where the hospital nurses and LC's assistance left off. Praise for the mothers who don't meet their breastfeeding dreams but move forward with resilience to embrace what is.

*The things that you are passionate about are not random,
they are your calling.*

- Fabienne Fredrickson

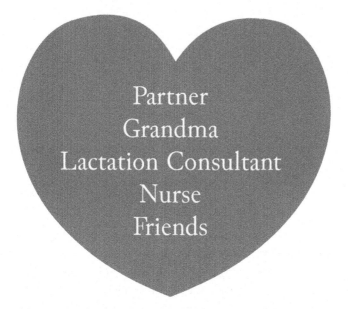

Partner
Grandma
Lactation Consultant
Nurse
Friends

One of the first LCs who joined our team recently turned 50. She lives across the country now. On this birthday, I had the occasion to tell her that she "had me at hello," right from the start. We had a preliminary phone interview before my boss's interview. The first thing she said to me after our introduction was, "I have a passion for breastfeeding." That's all I needed to hear. Maybe not all passions are meant to last a lifetime. Sometimes the field of lactation is a springboard for something else. It can be discouraging to lose LCs to other positions but be grateful for who is with you today, sharing your passion. Thank you for your passion, especially on the weary days.

Letting Go

The only person you're destined to become is the person you decide to be.

- Ralph W. Emerson

Your values shape your behavior, but on any given day, your behavior can also be caused by triggers. It's normal to have emotional reactions in certain situations. Thinking about one right now? If so, take a deep breath. Exhale. It's easy to reflect on the positive triggers: a latch (yeah!), support from a supervisor (gratitude), a kindness from a family member (joy), or less paperwork (over the moon!). We don't live in Mary Poppins' bubble, though, do we? You might be blamed for something that wasn't your fault, given more responsibilities on a given day than is reasonable, experience displaced anger from a mother, witness a colleague showing racial bias. We can stew over some events, lose sleep, let it impact our professional work, or try to control someone else. The path to inner peace may just be to let go. That doesn't necessarily mean inaction, but it does mean detachment. Ask for that grace. Then your actions and responses will be from a place of freedom.

We all have the extraordinary coded within us, waiting to be released.

- J. L. Houston

During the pandemic, many mothers have suffered the loss of their personal breastfeeding support network. This has given birth to creative ways to assure moms have the help they need. There are now more virtual consults being offered, webinars on telehealth, position statements on the safety of breastfeeding and keeping moms and babies together, and safe handling of human milk. Some of us may provide consults for patients in the hospital while fully gowned, gloved, and masked. It's hot in there! It's extraordinary to witness such generosity of spirit and self.

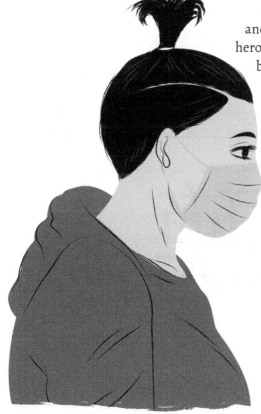

Everyone in one form or another puts on their super-hero cape and does their part but that cape comes off at the end of the day. You, too, may be exhausted, lonely, worried, sad, or financially vulnerable. I suspect there have been signs of PTSD in the healthcare community. Are you okay? How will you respond when your circle of support asks, "How can we help?"

Light

*(S)he would walk into my mind as if it were a town and
s(he) a torchlight procession of one lighting up the street.*

- Unknown

Who do you imagine when you read this epigraph? Likely, it's unrelated to lactation. A parent, sibling, partner, or childhood friend. Spend some quality moments with that image. What a gift to have someone so important to you that the thought of them lights up your life!

When challenge is present, the teacher is in the room.

- Unknown

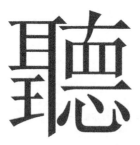

You, or someone you love, may be in a dark place right now. It's often in retrospect when lessons can be gleaned from struggles and suffering. Heaven knows many of us have companioned mothers who truly suffer through a breastfeeding experience. While we have an ethical commitment to stay with the mom in the moment, it's not easy to be present and unable to fix the situation. Still, we listen wholeheartedly; we empathize, and we sit in the silence of the non-answers because the need to be heard and understood is so vital to every human being. This Chinese character for listening aptly includes the symbol for hearing, mind, seeing, focusing, feeling, and being present! We are offering her the gift of ourselves. It will not go unappreciated, and it very well may be her saving grace.

Imprinting

Our first experience of life is primarily felt in the body.
Our mother's gaze is our first relational imprinting.
Her early mirroring stays with us our whole life. I am
sure that you have seen how mother and child fix on
each other with total delight during breastfeeding. It is
almost eucharistic. We know ourselves in the security of
those who love us and gaze upon us.

- Richard Rohr OFM, *Founder, Center for Action and*
Contemplation

I have been captivated by watching the *Netflix* series *Babies*. The breastfeeding relationship is so beautifully portrayed. What a gift you have been given to witness breastfeeding couplet interactions. We see a mom relax into the moment once her baby latches. Because her wellbeing is so critical to the baby's wellbeing, nurturing the mother and helping her assume her maternal role, even when the latch isn't achieved, is crucial. Beyond that, the series records skin-to-skin (STS) contact interactions. It's a gentle reminder to promote this among the adopting parents and those who opt not to breastfeed. It's the rare mother who hasn't imprinted the first contact with her newborn. She remembers. The mirroring goes both ways.

*I keep my ideals because, in spite of everything, I still
believe that people are really good at heart.*

- Anne Frank

Were you a first responder during the COVID-19 outbreak? Did you
self-quarantine for the sake of a specific loved one or simply for the
common good? I did. In fact, part of this book has been written
during the pandemic. Ten years ago, while in Amsterdam, we vis-
ited the home where Anne Frank hid. She, her family, and 3 others
sequestered in 450 square feet for 25 months. 25 months! I've been
home for 10 weeks, and even with that, I can take a walk, ride my bike,
FaceTime with family, and have Zoom meetups with friends. For me,
this pandemic has given rise to virtual consults with mothers, emails,
phone contacts, texts, and Zoom with a breastfeeding Facebook support group. Finding ways to engage with moms and provide help
and support has blossomed. All is not lost. There are reasons to be
grateful and continued reasons to reach out where you can.

Time

Ninety percent of life is just showing up.

- Woody Allen

Time can be an enemy of a good caregiver. It's impossible not to be conscious of the clock when you have mothers you are seeing back-to-back. There can be inadequate time to decompress or process what you may have experienced with one mom when you are popping right into the next consult. Still, you are obligated to keep moving. How do you refocus to be attentive to the next person? (Maybe that's applicable even within your family.)

Here are some tips I've found helpful: 1) Take a few moments to think about what your most important intervention will likely need to be, 2) Inhale and exhale a slow breath or two, 3) Keep eye contact with the mom. Moms tend to cue off of you. When she realizes, by your presence, that you've indeed "shown up" for her, she'll relax too and better communicate her and her baby's needs.

The only gift is a portion of thyself. The poet, his poem,
the painter, his picture, the shepherd, his lamb.

- Ralph Waldo Emerson, *Self-Reliance*

Today, my daughter-in-law sent me pictures of her childhood that included time spent in her grandparents' colorful flower and vegetable garden. I'm struck by the immense power of the images we carry from the past. The gift of a flower, the condolence card, or the person who gave us excellent care during a hospitalization. When you are confident about what your gifts are and share them generously with others, they are remembered. Sometimes it's a name, sometimes just a feeling a mom has when she thinks of who helped her. Don't be stingy with the gift of self. It returns to you 100-fold.

I was moved recently when reading Anne LaMott's book, *Halleluiah Anyway.* In it, she reminded me/us that in all those many years of child-raising, what was given; "this beauty is not lost, it cannot be. All that we gave remains."

Patience

Many cultures . . . cement a natural bias to be kindest to those they know best, through social courtesies, to assure harmonious relationships with those they interact with daily.

- Christina Gross-Loh, *Parenting without Borders:*
Surprising Lessons Parents Around the
World Can Teach Us

Someone once told me they were impressed with how patient I was with the nurses on the maternity ward. How could I be anything but when I count on them to care for the mother-baby pairs when I leave? I'm sure that, at times, I was unable to contain my frustration about [fill in the blank]. I'm equally sure that the staff could be frustrated with me, wanting gold-standard care for a breastfeeding couplet. At the same time, they may have a heavy patient load that includes a mother receiving blood or having hourly blood-pressure monitoring. Still, we were kind to each other because we needed each other. There are times when we are more acutely aware of our interdependence than others. Thank God for those times, lest we may forget our true place in the scheme of things.

In all affairs, it's a healthy thing now and then,
to hang a question mark on the things you have long
taken for granted.

- Bertrand Russell

How does mother-baby care move forward? Often, it's with a practice-oriented question. It was over a half-century ago that a nurse noticed that babies on the window side of the nursery were less jaundiced than those on the shaded side. She wondered if sunlight helped break down bilirubin? Fast forward, and another question was asked. Why are we separating mothers and babies? The questions are endless. They drive research, but they also drive shifts in our own practice. What is the percentage of insufficient milk supply in modern society? How soon should a baby be seen post-discharge? As more states legalize cannabis, what are the risks to the fetus and newborn? What are your questions? When do you find yourself thinking, "I disagree with that practice?" If you are an early questioner, it takes courage to speak up, doesn't it?

Responding to Cries

*And if you have children, when they cry, does it not stir
something deep inside you?*

- Victor Hugo, *The Hunchback of Notre Dame*

It's so gratifying when you place a baby skin to skin, and cries turn into bliss. Remember when the research came out showing that a baby's cortisol level is lower if allowed to nurse during a painful procedure such as a heel stick? Still, there are tears, wails, and moments of inconsolability, and it's not always the baby. Our nurturing side, so full of compassion, wants to rock them both. Sometimes it's moms who feel they have to try the "cry it out" method as part of the sleep routine. We can't always stop them. In fact, perhaps we've known folks who have used it, and within a few days, the baby is fast asleep in minutes. (Newer research has shown that they still have higher cortisol levels, though.) I may want to impose my garnered wisdom from experience and reading of the data: try safe breastsleeping (see James McKenna, *Safe Infant Sleep*) or try nursing them to sleep. But the trial and error we allowed ourselves as parents may have to suffice for the moms as well. Maternal sleep deprivation can wreak havoc on emotional stability, exclusive breastfeeding, the immune system, and relationships. We can't ignore potential collateral damage as we try our best to support the mother *where she is.*

The moment we cease to hold each other, the moment we break faith with one another, the sea engulfs us, and the light goes out.

- James Baldwin, *Nothing Personal*

There were times I sought supervision over what I considered a critical incident with a colleague or manager. It is so easy to think we've "let it go," as the Disney song says, just because the emotional reaction to the situation has passed. Maybe we've inserted an appropriate pause, considered our part in the miscommunication, and refrained from simply complaining to others. There is that next step, though. Doing whatever is appropriate to make sure we don't break faith with one another. It takes humility. Sometimes it takes speaking with a third party. Maybe this resonates with a past or current work situation. Maybe it resonates because of an encounter with someone significant in your life. Don't wait too long to attend to it. It's always worth the risk to be graciously transparent.

Influencing Change

We cannot tell what may happen to us in this strange
medley of life. But we can decide what happens in us,
how we take it, what we do with it – and that is what
really counts in the end.

- Joseph Fort Newton

Don't we all have gut reactions to things that happen to us and around us? Life is not based on fairness. What do we do with these truths? Why do bad things happen to good people? Why are decisions made or initiatives neglected that are counter to the good of the mothers we serve? Why is this [insert specific thing] happening to me? If it's the mothers we're talking about, I hope you find meaningful ways to influence change. Still, sometimes the only appropriate response is *"enough."* Hopefully, it will be well-considered and not a knee-jerk reaction, whether that be in the professional realm or personal sphere. "Enough" may mean walking away, but it may mean working for systemic changes or changes in long-held ways we respond verbally or emotionally to the same situation over and over.

When something is important enough, you do it even if the odds are not in your favor.

- Elon Musk

Well, Mr. Musk may "Endeavor" to get to outer space, but probably not most of us. But it does make me think of the oft used phrase, "I love you to the moon and back." What or who do we love enough to go "all the way," so to speak? Who comes with us on that journey? Does anything or anyone get left behind? Sometimes we mistakenly think no one (or the someone who matters) shares our commitment. Perhaps it's true, or perhaps in the list of the top 5 priorities, you rank your particular passion as first, while they rank that same passion as fifth. How each of you lives that passion can look vastly different, even though it made both of your top 5 lists of values.

WEEK 29 **Promoting Equity**

*Think occasionally of the suffering of which you spare
yourself the sight.*

- Albert Schweitzer

It's challenging to avoid the 24-hour news cycle in the 21st century. In the wake of pandemics and racism protests, it has become increasingly difficult to ignore the suffering. That can be a good thing. Just don't let it paralyze you from doing whatever your part is to alleviate it. Proximity matters. It fuels compassion, and hopefully, it fuels educating yourself and taking action as well. One of the things this moment in history has done is to expose the fault lines in societies, the inequities, and the pervasiveness of the impact of poverty on nearly every aspect of a person's life. Because breastfeeding is something of a leveler, your work to support moms promotes equity. What can you do? Maybe you're already doing it or maybe there's something more.

The value of life is revealed when it confronts death from close quarters.

- Apoorve Dubey

During the period of social distancing due to COVID-19, I committed to writing an ethical will. It was an idea prompted before the virus by a friend within my circle of spiritual companions. It's worth considering your values, hopes, and lessons learned. Your legacy will be more than just your occupation, and certainly more than your finances. What stories will be told by those who share about you in the future? Do the important people in your life know the values that matter to you – the ones that are the underpinning of so many decisions and responses to what you've confronted in your life? What matters most to you? What were your defining moments?

LOSS

*I didn't want to kiss you goodbye, that was the trouble;
I wanted to kiss you good night. And there's a lot of
difference.*

- Ernest Hemmingway

Denial, anger, bargaining, depression, acceptance – the well-known stages of grief as identified by Elizabeth Kubler-Ross. If you have been even adjacently involved in a parent's loss of a newborn, there is often no time to proceed so methodically through something so utterly catastrophic. You watch helplessly as a mother holds her preemie skin to skin one last time, or you witness her tears as you pass her when she's wheeling back from the intensive care unit, or you hear, after the fact, of a sudden infant death case of someone's newborn you'd only last week been helping to latch. It makes no sense.

My own daughter called when her firstborn was weeks old and told me she thought she understood the meaning of grace. She proceeded to say that her most fearful moments are those before she falls asleep. Then she awakens, and Ava is still breathing. "I think that's grace," she relayed. Of course, it is. You wish that you could give guarantees for every tomorrow, but you've seen enough of death that you can only hope. When a parent is stricken with an unexpected loss, you reach across the chasm of what was to what now is and embrace the loss with her—compassion and perhaps your own experiences of loss, your only guide.

30: LOSS

Regret is a sad, harsh feeling when we fail to do some-thing our heart wanted to do.

- Anurag Prakash Ray

Have you heard friends say that they don't want to live with any regrets? This seems to compel them forward, but living with regrets and having regrets are two different things. Living with them implies you haven't let them go. Having them implies that you're human. Not everything works out – not for us, nor for our families. It is a sad thing when a mother decides she has to close the door to her nursing experience or desire for a breastfeeding experience. I've seen enough moms come to peace with their decisions that I can counsel other moms that surely, they too will get through the loss. It may be the only option left. It may be the right decision, and you can help her see the bigger picture and offer perspective. But—and I think it's a big but—don't avoid acknowledging the loss and disappointment. She may not understand why this outcome was part of her journey in life. These are soul questions for her to grapple with. But we know that the way she honors her heart is naming the loss.

59

Relationships

> *My work as a lactation consultant intertwines with my life outside the hospital, creating a tapestry of relationships that begin in unexpected places.*
>
> - Chris Auer, *Under One Sky*

I was leaving a Bed and Breakfast in Ireland in 2018 when the host learned of my profession. Immediately, she began to share the joys and struggles of her own breastfeeding journeys with her two sons. Ireland does not have the best breastfeeding initiation and duration rates. This mom made it 18 months for both. This was her goal. Still, when she saw other moms nursing older babies, she had pangs of regret for "only" going 18 months. She asked, "What do you think? Should I have kept going?" A year after weaning the youngest, she is still asking for reassurance.

The year prior, I walked the loop around the lake at the county park, blocks from our home. I overheard two African American moms discussing breastfeeding as they strolled with their babies. Several yards past them, I returned to ask how motherhood was going. The babies were 1 month old, the same age as my granddaughter, Olivia. Every 2 months, we seemed to find each other on the path and swap notes. We aren't always the educators. Moms teach us if we welcome them into our world.

There's much talk in our society about motherhood in general, but an awkward silence surrounds many of the concrete realities.

- Trudelle Thomas, *Spirituality in the Mother Zone*

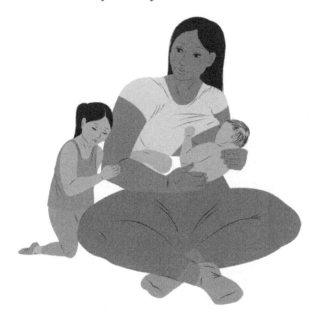

The 10th step of the Baby-Friendly Hospital Initiative is to refer moms to breastfeeding resources post-discharge. I am happy to say that some of these venues are the very places where the silence is broken, and moms can share frankly about the "mother zone." One such place is the Baby Café (currently in a virtual format during the pandemic). Another may be private breastfeeding moms' Facebook groups. Perhaps not all of these are as welcoming and open as the Southwest Ohio Breastfeeding Moms group of which I'm a part. It's refreshing to hear moms share with such transparency about issues from postpartum depression to being primarily bottle-feeders to strategies that help them negotiate conversations with their parents who aren't on the same page. Social media can be a gift.

Wings

There are only two lasting bequests we can give our children: one is roots and the other is wings.

- Johann Wolfgang von Goethe

At the beginning of a parenting journey, these words can be romantically sweet. When you are further down the parenting road, you intuit, then experience, the lived reality of those words. They go from being romantic to bittersweet to sometimes just plain sad. They are true, and there is a sorrow to the implications of such closure. Spend a few minutes considering how these words strike you.

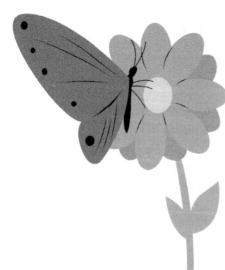

As breastfeeding advocates, the words may hold different meanings. Moms who couldn't thank us enough with their firstborns may need little to nothing from us with subsequent babies. The bond isn't broken; the moms have wings now. You were a part of that! Good on ya, as the Aussies say.

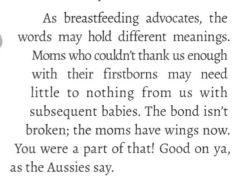

A baby is God's opinion that the world should go on.

- Carl Sandburg

It's been reported that if the 2020 pandemic lockdown goes on for 6 months (into the fall of 2020), there could be upwards of 7 million babies born in the coming 2021. Who's surprised at that? We, in this field, may have more work cut out for us. What joy these little ones give us! Such a gift to meet the gaze of one who has come so fresh from God.

Person-First

> *Yet isn't it in this inner realm where mothers really*
> *live – facing unfamiliar waves of anxiety, desire, and*
> *uncertainty that accompany each day with a new*
> *baby?... New mothers often wonder whether others are*
> *going thru a similar upheaval.*

> - Daniel & Nadia Stern,
> Pediatrician & Psychiatrist, *Birth of a Mother*

Might you need to review your own self-talk, that brain chatter that makes you feel this *one* issue is yours alone? No one else could possibly be experiencing it. Does it feel too embarrassing or too trivial to share with a trusted companion? If so, then you can empathize with what mom may be vocalizing to you.

Shame and self-doubt can keep any of us from asking for validation. Being proactive and giving the mom a safe space to verbalize her concerns can never be replaced by a suggestion for an app. The chances are that whatever she's experiencing, there are another dozen moms in your city or town who are in the same space. Letting her know that she's not alone can result is a huge sense of relief. Don't forget to refer her to mom groups. You don't have to save everyone.

But getting back to your self-talk. Share your story with someone who's earned the right to hear it. You're worth it.

The human spirit is one of ability, perseverance, and
courage that no disability can steal away.

- Unknown

The moment I heard a young man say that he didn't have a disability (clearly, he did), it "just took him longer," I knew that all would be fine in his future. For new moms, their baby can't give them that reassurance. Issues that may arise because of a history of extreme prematurity or a well-known diagnosis may have indeterminant outcomes. What can you do? It begins with how you communicate. Using "person-first" language lets a mom know you see her baby as a whole person, not just a disability. To say, "I'm taking care of the Down's baby in room 24" isolates the newborn to one category and indirectly encourages others to see her through that solitary lens. It inadvertently introduces a bias in expectations. The alternative: "I'm taking care of a baby with Down syndrome." Perhaps we don't all have disabilities, but we all have our Achilles heel and look at us; thriving despite it. What a wonderful gift you give new parents when you model seeing the whole baby!

Great Love

You are okay. You will get better. You will feel yourself again. You may not believe that's possible now: Cling to it anyway.

- Unknown

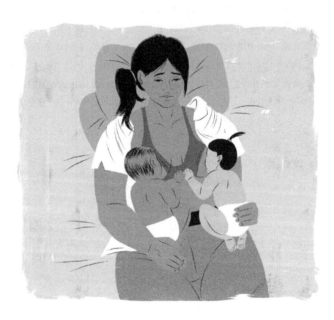

There are several risk factors for postpartum depression, some of which we may be able to identify during the pregnancy if we happen to be in a setting where we interact with moms prenatally. Even then, if your setting doesn't use a risk-assessment tool, you may not be prompted to ask. Here are a few factors that should sound familiar:

family history, psychosocial factors that involve her significant other, birthing multiples, history of difficulty with breastfeeding, seasonal depression, prior history of substance abuse, poor social support, no partner involvement, unplanned pregnancy, history of anxiety or postpartum depression, illness (diabetes, thyroiditis), and stressful (traumatic) event in the pregnancy. Additional post-birth factors include delivery by cesarean section (USA average is 31.9% as of 2018 data), premature birth, or the birth of a baby with an illness.

While this is not an exhaustive list, you may be exhausted reviewing it. How can this topic lead you to a peaceful reflection today? I hope it does because recognizing a mother in need, or in potential future need, is key to meeting her not only body but mind and spirit. This epigraph by an unknown author is such a beautiful way to reassure a mother. It is worth repeating to her more than once. When all is dark, and if added to that, there is guilt over not feeling enthralled with her newborn, it's hard for a mom, or anyone for that matter, to envision that she will feel herself again. Early identification is crucial, first, because she's suffering, and second, because the earlier the intervention, the better and the sooner she'll be feeling her version of okay. When a mother can't believe this, believe it for her.

Perhaps you can be present in this way because you've experienced postpartum depression, anxiety, or psychosis. But maybe it's just because you've known dark days or even weeks. Maybe you are there right now: a significant loss, a life-event, or something said by someone you love triggers your insecurities. You find yourself thinking, "Who I am is wrong." Or maybe you're ashamed of something that happened or something you said or did.

Who or what is your anchor while you ride these emotional waves? They always pass. You know they do. But knowing that may not help until some lightness of being descends upon you, almost by grace: a serenity, a word of comfort, the gift of detachment, or a memory. The anchor seems less needed because hope is born.

None of us, including me, ever do great things. But we
can all do small things with great love, and together we
can do something wonderful.

- Mother Theresa

Some in the lactation field have become known worldwide through their research, writing, or speaking. Maybe the number is amped up a bit due to social media platforms. Still, it is relatively uncommon to have notoriety. But, as the woman of Calcutta reminds us, we can do small things with great love. I believe that the vast majority of us are capable of doing small things with great love. In fact, I think we're already doing it, hidden and daily though it may be. But who needs recognition? We are living our "something wonderful" on most days. That is its own reward. By its hidden nature, we can miss the beauty of it. Pause and take it in. You know when your presence to a mother has been the most important gift of her day. Take it in. Bless yourself for your generosity. If you work with a team, acknowledge to one another that together, you are doing something wonderful. Teams need that validation as well.

Perspective

It is an absolute human certainty that no one can know his own beauty, or perceive a sense of his (or her) own worth, until it has been reflected back to him (her) in the mirror of another loving, caring human being.

- J. J. Powell

We are this sacred space for mothers, giving them the clarity that, above all else, is their love for their child. When feeding frenzies have her pulling her hair out, we remind her she is the mirror. Give her perspective. When she's sleep-deprived and at her wit's end, remind her that she is her baby's mirror. The most important thing is not the feeding outcome. Even when she's successful, this too shall pass. Okay, maybe she won't wean until age 7. Still, it will pass. What won't pass is her need to see her worth, regardless of the outcome. What can you mirror today that allows someone to know their beauty? I hope this book, while not a mirror, reminds you that there are many people who value you. There is a famous image called "Trinity" by Russian iconographer Andrei Rublev. History tells us it is the depiction of the three angels that appeared to Abraham. There is a small rectangular empty space at the front of the table where they sit. Some say that Rublev originally placed an object there that was made to be mirror-like, perhaps tin. So, the observer is introduced into the divine image as part of the story. We, too, are part of the story of many families. Where do you see yourself playing your part?

A thousand threads connect us, and among those fibers,
as sympathetic threads, our actions run as causes, and
they come back to us as effects.

- Herman Melville

Navajo blankets usually have an error interwoven into them intentionally. A little humble reminder that no one is perfect; therefore, nothing is perfect either. Sometimes our actions, whether conversations or interventions, are at least near-perfect. We help a mother place her baby prone on her belly, and *Voila!* He roots his way to her and self-attaches.

Often, we don't get to see the long-term outcomes of our efforts because the mother's journey has moved on. We might learn later that the effect was not as we intended. She struggled at home alone, or she misunderstood the instruction we thought we'd so clearly conveyed. Nothing is perfect, and there are consequences. Even so, there are times we hear the final chapter of her story months or even years later. The story may come back to us in a heart-warming manner; it worked, after all. If you call to mind any of these stories today, whisper a thank you.

Wisdom

Discernment is the choice between two goods.

\- Spirituality of Ignatius of Loyola

Consider this quote in light of the "art" of human-milk feeding. There may be more than one path to offer a mother to reach her goal. You may have more than one trick up your sleeve. Sometimes though, the pending decision is bigger than an approach. Sometimes it's not even about the act of breastfeeding or pumping. Sometimes you are helping her find her own wisdom.

Sometimes you are searching for wisdom yourself. What's the next phase of my journey, and how will I get there? Discernment is bigger than weighing the pros and cons. Perhaps you even find yourself making the proverbial 2-column list. But when listening whole-heartedly, don't you find it helpful to be attentive to your sense of peace or anxiety and to where you are drawn or feel hesitant? Time can be a gift during important decision-making periods. It allows you to notice your feelings and intuitions as you consider various possibilities.

It would be easier if everything were black and white, good and bad. Who wouldn't choose good? But discernment is more about looking at what is best among valid other options. Be patient with the process, and when possible, don't burn bridges.

There is no such thing as a baby. There is only a baby and someone.

- D. J. Winnicott

Dependent, dependent, dependent. Compare us to any other mammal or even primate, for that matter; you just won't find any newborn more helpless. We've all done milk content comparisons and know that the lower fat content, coupled with the fact that we aren't a nesting species, means moms hold and feed human babies often.

I chuckle when I read James McKenna citing studies that show during the night; breastfed babies feed more often and more minutes compared to bottle-feeding counterparts. This alone could not be a marketing tool for breastfeeding. However, when he explains the value of frequent arousals at night as a means of decreasing the risk of SIDS, you can't help but appreciate our biology and its unique mechanisms to keep our young safe. Still, do you ever feel a bit squirmy about how to a) educate a pregnant mom so she can anticipate frequent night-time feedings and appreciate why they happen, or b) support the mom in the throes of fatigue with no respite at night? We know it's a phase, but there's no telling how long an individual baby will be up 2-3 times per night.

If we could only give them the end-date. It's challenging to be transparent on this topic partly because the stance of the American Academy of Pediatrics (AAP) on safe sleep is a one-size-fits-all statement and doesn't give us permission to address what is safe in the context of a particular family. Until there are more evidence-based guidelines coming from the professional organizations, we have to, at the least, promote close proximity at night and remind moms that "there is only a baby and someone."

Courage

We cultivate love when we allow our most vulnerable and powerful selves to be deeply seen and known and when we honor the spiritual connection that grows from that offering with trust, respect, kindness, and affection.

- Brené Brown

On our academic career pathway, we've all been educated on the importance of keeping a professional distance and maintaining boundaries. Likely, we've been on the receiving end of a parent disclosing themselves with amazing transparency. Examples: A mother's doubts, her ambivalence, or her worries (or his worries). It takes courage to share on that level.

Perhaps there have also been circumstances where, quite appropriately, you have been transparent in return. I don't mean repeating what the chills after an epidural were like for you. I mean sharing a similar moment of pain, doubt, sadness – more as living proof that she is not alone. I hope you are fortified by moments like this with a friend or loved one. Whatever situation arises that allows this level of intimacy, welcome it as a gift of trust that you have received or given. All experiences of being at one with, are expressions of grace.

Love is an intention and an action.- Scott Peck, *The Road Less Traveled*

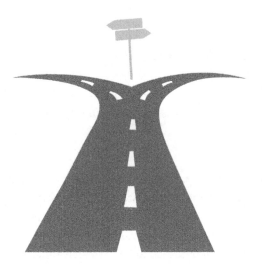

In our fairytale childhoods, it was enough for love to be a romantic intention. Stage one was the honeymoon phase. The baby, the beloved, or the new job couldn't be more wonderful. Then things start to get serious. We are up more than expected with the baby. Something is being asked of us that heretofore had not been in the relationship mix. There's a bit of disillusionment added to the bliss. Now we are on the threshold of committed love.

With newborns having the "cute factor," nature has given them the means to help create permanent attachment. But with our beloved or our beloved career, not so instinctual when the going gets rough, is it? What keeps you committed? How does that show itself in outward action? The transitory feelings of love can be just that, transitory. We rely on our inner wisdom and values to shape our decisions. How would someone else describe your love in action? Love is not easy. No wonder it's considered the road less traveled.

Gratitude

Let us swim together in the ocean of our being.

- Jonathan Lockwood Huie

Think about a mother's expression of gratitude directed toward you. It's not the thank-you of providing an extra blanket she's requesting. It's more profound, isn't it? You have no doubt that it's deeply heartfelt. She has received something from you even beyond the latch or pumping support. What is it that has affected her so profoundly? I think she intuits that you have crossed the ocean to reach her. You've met her at the soul level that recognizes your presence as a guide, listener, advocate, comforter, and empowerer (okay, not a word, but you get what I mean). Your very person was the gift that went beyond your offer of expertise, and she didn't even have to ask for it.

I hope you experience that in return, through your network of peers, your chat groups, your social network, or your family. It takes more than a bit of vulnerability to ask for what you need. Ask.

We learn from the gardens to deal with the most urgent question of the time: How much is enough?

- Wendell Berry

How long do you recommend breastfeeding? Do you use the WHO guideline of 2 years, the AAP guide of 1 year (or longer, as mutually desired)? Do you roll with what the mom says? When moms have said so happily that they plan to nurse for 2 weeks, you know they've likely heard something about colostrum being mixed with mature milk through 2 weeks. You educate, you validate, you encourage, but she will ultimately have to be the one to decide what is enough. During a recent virtual breastfeeding moms meeting, a mother of a 15-month old who is exclusively breastfed mentioned as an aside that she'd have weaned before now. Still, their pediatric allergist recommended nursing for 2 years. Her son was diagnosed with a dairy and egg allergy at 5 months of age, and she was told this increased his risk of acquiring asthma by 50%. Mentioning that, while breastfeeding is no panacea, it does decrease the risk of asthma; she and the other moms on Zoom all said this was news to them. This is even more surprising because we live in the Ohio River Valley and have high rates of asthma. At one point, our region had the largest number of specialists in the country addressing pediatric asthma. You may have your pet items you convey when you speak about the benefits of breastfeeding. It helps to ask a bit about family health history. It can be exponentially more powerful to be able to target your education, so she's making the decision through a wider lens.

Maternity Leave

Oh, how the heart approaches what it yearns.

\- Paul Simon, songwriter

Have you companioned mothers who are approaching the end of their maternity leave? So many are asking for a sympathetic ear as they try to envision and prepare for what it will be like to go back to a full-time position and maintain their breastfeeding relationship. Whether it be 3 weeks or 3 months or something in between, it's not the logistics of it; it's the heart yearning for "just a little more time," affordable daycare, and more freedom to choose.

Often, the day arrives while their baby is still up 2-3 times at night. We can talk strategies all we want, but what many mothers want is to have longer paid maternity leave without the fear of losing their job. While the 1993 US Family Medical Leave Act guarantees 12 weeks after birth, there is no stipulation of being paid. Fewer than half of the private-sector workers are eligible for this leave.

During a visit to the largest maternity hospital in Europe in 2018, I saw something quite different. Parents get 480 days paid leave in Sweden (the UK 280 days with 90% pay). The only countries that do not mandate paid leave are Lesotho, Swaziland, and Papua New Guinea. How did the U. S. end up on *that* list?

The US Lactation Consultant Association (USLCA) keeps American LCs abreast of pending legislation and encourages us to contact legislators to support better maternity leave laws. I know it's hard to add this to seeing mothers, tending to your own life, and getting involved with the legislation. Only you know what you can handle but take a moment to ponder it. Our professional organizations can't keep saying exclusive breastfeeding is the gold standard and then watch as the rug is pulled out from under a mom during the critical early months.

Invisible threads are the strongest ties.

- Friedrich Nietzsche

Mister Rogers is known for encouraging people to look for the helpers. You need not look further than your own mirror. Consider, where do the threads of connection branch out from you? Families, of course. Which families? Some LCs remark that their favorite moms to work with are those with babies in the NICU; others with mom's returning to work before 8 weeks; still others with the poor, or Black, or Appalachian, or immigrants, yet others, with mothers in addiction recovery. In each of these mom's life experiences, we see minorities. Anywhere threads connect, we are bound to experience mutuality. It knows no racial, gender, or socioeconomic limits. The joy of threads connecting us to the underserved or those who have added suffering is boundless. Widening our hearts to be inclusive of the marginalized widens our capacity for compassion and constructively addresses disparities in breastfeeding rates.

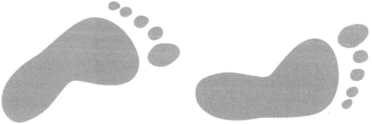

Handholding

Sometimes reaching out and touching someone's hand is the beginning of a journey.

- Vera Nazarian

Today, I am instant messaging a mom in Ecuador, the very mom I'd Skyped with, then written about when using this epigraph in *Under One Sky*. I am commenting on a caricature of life with a baby and toddler that she's posted on Facebook. I ask her to consider joining a Baby Café virtual gathering to talk about her experiences. For all its legitimate disadvantages, the internet does allow us to reach out and touch someone, albeit virtually.

No matter the type of consult, while we were handholding, let's remember that *our* hand was being held as well. Sometimes the day goes by too quickly to linger on what that touch meant. The twilight hours may provide those moments, maybe even as you read this. Some of those with whom we interact leaves fingerprints on our hearts. Did she have something to teach you? Is it a lesson that keeps recycling for you because you've yet to learn the lesson? What about her touched you? Did it trigger a distant memory? Can you savor that at this moment?

Instead of growing in my belly, they grew in my heart.

- Anonymous

Recently reading from Hoda Katb's book, *I Really Needed This Today*, she quotes her daughters, who say, "We grew in momma's heart." The sentiment is the same. What is not organic becomes organic because of the heart. It's a beautiful and honest way to see adoption. Whether it applies to children or other connections that transcend blood, may we each celebrate the truth that seeing with the eyes of the heart connects us with some pretty wonderful human beings.

Hearing

When a woman is talking to you, listen to what she says with her eyes.

- Victor Hugo

We too, as women, can be guilty of listening without hearing, whether it's to a mom, a fellow provider, a boss, a colleague, a partner, our child, or our adult child. Women may not have the corner market on communicating with their eyes, but, especially if you're intuitive, you pick up that those eyes of a new mother do tell a story.

What are you picking up? An unspoken heartbreak or a home worry? Sometimes they may appear to be putting on a brave face when you see exhaustion written everywhere. Now what? How we respond may, in part, be based on how much time we have to dive in. Sometimes the wise listener knows not to dive in. The only exception to that rule will be if you suspect that she's a victim of some level of violence. Then we rely on both her eyes and your gut feeling, followed by some means of validating. A gentle and private approach or referral to a social worker is in order. We all long to be seen and heard, even when we're not talking.

Don't waste your time dividing the world into the good
guys and the bad guys. Hold them both together in your
own soul – where they are anyway – and you will have
held together the whole world. You will have overcome
the great divide in one place of spacious compassion.

- Richard Rohr, *Everything Belongs*

In the hospital setting, while infrequent, we care for incarcerated mothers who've delivered. It may not be as overt for you in your practice setting, but do you ever find yourself dividing folks into "those like me, and everyone else?" Or the gay and straight, or the wed and unwed, or the legal and the undocumented? The list is endless when we seek to separate ourselves. Rohr says it succinctly; "the good guys and the bad guys."

When we can identify with some aspect of a mother's backstory, barriers between us begin to fade, and true companionship is a real possibility. An amazing grace is when we can open ourselves to who she is, in all her strengths and weaknesses, even when we know nothing of her backstory. The gift for mom is that we now have the strongest possibility of influencing her motherhood path. The gift for us is enlarging our humanity.

Generosity

*Victor Frankl wrote that human beings create meaning
in three ways: through their work, through their
relationships, and how they choose to meet unavoidable
suffering. Every life brings hardship and trial, and
every life also offers deep possibilities for meaningful
work and love . . . I've learned that courage and
compassion are two sides of the same coin.*

- Eric Greitens, *The Warrior's Heart*

As I write, the world is in the early stages of its first reopening
after the initial COVID-19 lockdown. I wonder how you're doing?
How are you coping? It certainly has created some suffering, both the
illness and the self-quarantine of those of us who are healthy. After
ten weeks of seeing no one, a friend recently came out for a 1-hour
masked visit on my porch. She confided that she and her husband
had missed 7 family celebrations (birthdays, anniversaries, Mother's
Day). It gets lonely out there, even if you have one house companion.
Was it avoidable? Technically, that answer could be "yes." We could
have ignored the orders and gone on with our gatherings, but the
Common Good called for something else. It took restraint, courage,
and a willingness to bear some of the load by not exposing ourselves
to our families and close friends.

I suppose there's no such thing as pure motivation. There was
likely some fear going into our decisions. Still, I'm wondering what
the meaning of your sacrifice was. Honestly, isn't there something
altruistic, something holy about it all?

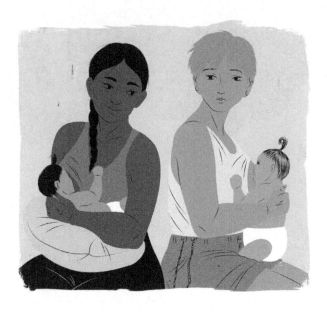

Even after all this time the sun never says to the earth,
"You owe me." Look what happens with a love like that, it
lights up the whole sky.

- Hafiz

During the pandemic, I have been participating in the Facebook group *View from My Window*. Within a few weeks, members totaled 2.3 million. People are hungry for connection. From the beautiful to the mundane, I've seen the views from members' windows. Reading the short stories that the writer includes affords the opportunity for an outpouring of compassion. Some are nurses on the frontline sharing pictures outside their New York hotels, some tell of the death of a spouse, parent, sibling, and some celebrate their birthday alone but with the group. They offer a bulwark against despair and isolation. Posts so often include what the person is thankful for and words of encouragement, despite some dire circumstances. We are truly living this *Under One Sky*.

84

In the online breastfeeding support group I'm a part of, there are two moms who have provided milk for others: over 5,200 ounces and 2,500 ounces, respectively. The former mom shipped this staggering volume to Prolacta, the other, to the Ohio Mother's Milk Bank. Both moms had babies in Level 3 NICU settings who underwent various surgeries in their first year of life. The first mom opted to sell the milk because she had no idea what costs her baby's medical needs would incur. She donates a huge part of her time to helping and supporting other mothers. Her milk has provided the substrate for human milk fortifier for 12 micro-preemies. The latter mom was an overproducer; a NICU nurse mentioned in passing that she might consider donating some of her milk. While having previously breastfed other babies, both continue to pump exclusively. Their cuties are now 15 and 10 months, respectively.

Think of the breadth of the impact of those choices for so many babies they'll never meet. I know we want to provide guidance for the overproducers to minimize the risk of plugs, mastitis, or abscesses. Still, consider remembering to tell moms about another option, even as they downshift supply.

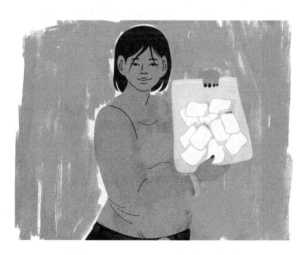

Give a little pause today as you consider the generosity of the mothers, you know. I hope you have a chance to affirm them. They are light in a sometimes-dark sky for families of preemies.

Honest Conversations

In each of our interactions we begin to realize there is something benevolent in the other that helps us let down our defenses and defensiveness.

- Richard Rohr, *Immortal Diamond*

As the United States is experiencing an eruption of protests after the death of an unarmed Black man, we see other countries marching in solidarity as well. Police reform and an end to mass incarceration are only part of the solution. We know from maternity data that Black women are 3-4 times more likely to die surrounding childbirth and 60% more likely to have premature births. What can one person do? It may begin with a dropping of our own guard to see differently. It may take an honest look at where implicit bias has been operative within us, within our community, and within our institution. Maybe you can consider donating to Peer Lactation Supporters of Color. We can't do everything, but there are probably several things we can do. I will always remember the reply of a Senegalese mother when I asked her what brought her to the U. S.; "Sometimes, life requires you to do things you didn't plan to do." Could this be your time, or my time?

Tell me and I forget, teach me and I may remember,
involve me and I learn.

- Benjamin Franklin

Might you consider this the next time a mother tells you she hasn't told the pediatrician where her baby sleeps at night? The way to safely sleep, presuming no risk factors, has been enumerated in great detail by James McKenna in his latest book, *Safe Infant Sleep*. His research, and that of others, seem to indicate that mothers aren't telling their providers what decision they made once they gathered all the facts. How sad.

If we encourage mothers to involve them, providers will have a much better understanding of what's happening in their practice and reconsider how to help parents make this decision based on their family circumstances. We know, and they know, that the greatest risk for SIDS is among the babies whose moms are under the influence of drugs (post-c-section narcotics or illicit), alcohol, and nicotine. Let's give moms encouragement to involve, and perhaps educate their doctor in this important conversation.

Partners

My soul has grown deep like the river.

- Langston Hughes

Silence and reflection invite the soul to plumb the depths, reconciling issues from the past, preparing you for what lies ahead and what's immediately before you. Feed your soul with both. How do you stop the brain chatter? Breathe. And again. And again. Sit a few minutes and ground your deepest self with the river.

Breathe

Partners have the key role of teaching the baby that love sometimes comes without food.

- LLL International, *The Womanly Art of Breastfeeding*

Don't you love this reminder hidden in plain sight? We can forget the obvious. There was a meeting in 2012 among care providers, nursing, and lactation staff, that focused on the evidence surrounding a change of practice in the entire city. Babies would be placed on mothers' chest immediately after birth, for one hour, or until the first breastfeeding. The hand of a young male neonatologist shot up. "But what about the father?" He was a dad himself. He related that this would be hard for fathers. It is a deferred need a partner commits to for the sake of the baby's wellbeing. I hope we can empower all partners to see the significance of their role. They aren't left out when we help them lean in, literally and figuratively.

Sacred Circle

You don't have to give birth to someone to have a family.
We're all family – extended family.

\- Sandra Bullock

Will you pause today to consider who your extended family is? Beyond aunts, uncles, nieces, and nephews, who is in your Sacred Circle? Who is on the margins of the Circle despite being in your life? Is there someone new you might include if you're able to widen your heart?

From my point of view, your life is already a miracle of
chance waiting for you to shape its destiny.

- Toni Morrison

I have often, with a bit of melancholy, said aloud, "I shall not pass this way again." From 1996 to 2019, I suffered from 10-12 migraines per week. I never left work, though you might find me vomiting in the nursery sink if I couldn't get to the restroom fast enough. Home by 6 pm, I lost the next 5 hours holed up in a dark bedroom. Add that up over a month, and it may be 60 hours I would never get back. My chance miracle was finally hitting on the right medicine.

When you have an obstacle, your life might not seem like a miracle. You may be unable to shape your destiny. You may feel constrained, disempowered, or unsupported. What's one action you can take today to express your belief in yourself? I hope a wonderful life awaits you. As the song says, "I hope you have the time of your life."

Dreams

Friends are kind to each other's hopes. They cherish each other's dreams.

- Henry David Thoreau

No matter how comfortable you are being alone with yourself, no matter how introverted you are, we all need community. We engage with folks in work, school, neighborhood, church, or sports. We may live with someone(s). We may have a plethora of friends or a single friend. Whenever we are with another person and feel safe, there we have a community. This is where we dare to share our personal dreams and listen to the dreams of others. Sometimes, life allows us to listen to the communal dream.

Each day, we are invited to live in solidarity with others. It gives us the gift of valuing other's dreams. We hear them in the mothers and families we serve. We listen to their sacred stories and affirm their dreams as important and worthy. Here's to experiencing this in reciprocity.

Each person is born with a defining image.

- James Hillman

I heard a speaker recently answer the question about what you should do when you're feeling disconnected from a person or group whose ideas are different than your own. She replied by suggesting that we learn the names and songs of 25 different birds. Instead of thinking that she sidestepped the question and the dilemma it speaks of, what she said seems to offer us a Zen koan. What do you think she meant? I wonder if it's tied into recognizing the defining image. If we can begin to appreciate the differences in the natural world, perhaps we can begin to appreciate the differences in others. If we can do that, we can approach each mother, patient, client, and colleague from a place that recognizes each person carries light and is indeed born with a defining image if we but posture ourselves to recognize it.

Normal Days

Normal day, let me be awake to the treasure you are.

- Mary Jean Irion

For many of us, there is a bit of a Groundhog Day experience in our daily routines at work, including our tasks and what we say to mothers. Would you say that most of your days are not out of the ordinary? Still, so many days hold a moment of beauty, or wonder, or something or someone that elicits gratitude. Hopefully, you had a good night's sleep and can be awake to receive.

A mosaic is a conversation between what is broken.

- T. T. Williams

Having spent more time at home as of late, I've seen some awesome chalk art that imitates stained-glass. This is another gift of isolation that the children have used to brighten the world. It reminds me of the beauty of the stained-glass windows in the church where I was married. There are dozens, each depicting a part of Jesus' journey on earth. When you look at only one frame, you don't have the advantage of seeing the whole story that's portrayed.

I think this is art imitating life. Whatever moment of life you're in now isn't the whole picture. Even if you are in a space of perfect contentment, it's a slice of your life. It may be more important to recall this, though, when things seem broken – a relationship, career path detour, a serious illness, a sadness that knows no words, or the world itself.

Caring for moms can be a good distraction when the soul is heavy. It may just open up your heart space to allow that conversation between what is broken so that something lovely and good and true can come of it. Trust the process.

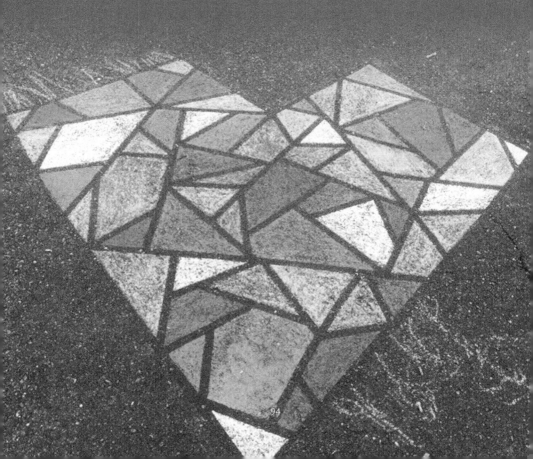

Pause

Insert a pause. - Theresa Horan Sapunar

I spoke too soon. (I've said that more than I care to admit.) I'm a slow learner. Each day gives us the chance to begin again. To be present. To be a better listener. A person's need to feel heard supersedes the need for answers that they may not even be asking you to provide. Yet, the common temptation for anyone in a caring profession is so often to "fix it." It's part of our training and part of our DNA, hence the restraint required to insert a pause has to be conscious. The gift it gives is so worth the effort that it takes to practice, fail, and practice more. It is transformative at work, in relationships, with children, and with adult children. You will not regret working hard to improve. Start now. Take a breath and collapse into your true self. Breathe again.

The 16 million children born in the wealthy countries will have 4X's the impact on the earth's resources than the 109 million born in the poor world.

- UNICEF

When you are with a specific mom at a specific moment, it's not likely that you're thinking about the bigger picture of how breastfeeding is better for the earth's natural resources. I don't often hear this touted to pregnant mothers, but let's remember that it's eco-friendly. Breastfeeding doesn't emit any greenhouse gases. It doesn't add to the local landfill. There are zero food miles involved from production to eating locally. You're mobilizing a generation that will help save the planet. That's something to smile about!

Life Force

I think that I shall never see a poem as lovely as a tree. A tree whose hungry mouth is pressed against the earth's sweet flowing breast.

- Joyce Kilmer

Am I the only one who has repeated the first sentence of this beloved poem, not realizing the metaphor that followed? Good grief. How did I miss that? What gorgeous imagery it conjures. Many of us are privileged to hold babies daily, hug them even. Let's at least metaphorically hug a tree today. Stop. Look out the window or turn the podcast off during your exercise routine. Find a tree and follow its trunk to the good earth's sweet flowing breast.

In the same way, trees fill our environment with oxygen, so nursing offers a child an essential lifeforce. Here, you are a party to it. Nelson Henderson said that "the true meaning of life is to plant a tree under whose shade you do not expect to sit." With rare exceptions, we won't see these babies grow into adulthood but we have helped plant a seed of health and bonding that will be that child's foundation. Kudos.

When the student is ready, the teacher will arise.

- Buddha

It's too bad about hindsight. Why does it have to be retrospective? Even with the understanding gained via hindsight, there are some errors we seem destined to repeat. Are there interventions you never use or referrals you'd never make because they don't make sense to you, but then a mother tells you it was exactly what fixed her feeding problem? Adjusting a palate, a frenotomy procedure, or laid-back breastfeeding. The list goes on. We reason that case studies are not population-based studies or randomized control trials, and we dismiss them. Twenty-seven years as a board-certified lactation consultant and moms are still teaching me not to be dismissive, not to be so "positive" about my position.

Then there are the moms. You hear from a mom you helped, and she's telling you about advice she's following, and you wonder why she couldn't hear it the first time you made the same recommendation. We all have our rhythm for receptivity to new ideas. The important thing is that she eventually heard it, even if we weren't the vehicle for the information.

All shall be well, and all shall be well, and all manner of things shall be well.

- Julian of Norwich

All Will Be Well

Why did this obscure English woman of the 14th century feel the need to repeat herself 3 times? Julian is the author of the oldest book written in English by a woman. Maybe she had pushback. Maybe she had to tell herself this repeatedly. She lived a cloistered life in a small building attached to a church, yet she wasn't isolated. She had a window open to the courtyard. People would come day and night to seek wisdom, tell their troubles, and ask for prayers. When you hear enough stories, perhaps you become grounded in something deeper than your current crisis. Maybe underneath the loss, the pain, and the suffering, there is a realm where your own peace cannot be touched. Maybe this was what she tried to communicate to her followers.

While this applies to all of us, it may be something important to convey to mothers when things aren't going as expected. No one can guarantee outcomes. You can be confident that underneath the situation is a benevolent force assuring us that all will be well. Companioning her is part of the way you embody trust in that ancient phrase.

Every doorway, every intersection, has a story.

- Kathleen Dunn

Today a mother told me that she blamed her baby's poor sleep on her mother. The baby's grandma had told the mom that she too was a poor sleeper, and Grandma hoped that one day her daughter would have to contend with what she dealt with as a young mother. Yikes! I hope that was said in jest. Still, I think it's true that our story begins with our mothers. They and partners are the doorway of this little one's life.

It's not uncommon for us to recycle experiences in adult life that harken back to our childhood. We may be triggered by a mother's birth experience that was similar to our own, especially if something traumatic happened. It gives us a lens as well as empathy. We are in a position to be part of the healing process. Sometimes we are with a mother during a second pregnancy and find her preemptively worrying that she'll have another bad experience. We are at the intersection of her journey for a reason. We can let her tell her story, which itself is healing. We may be in a position to advocate, to give anticipatory guidance, to refer her – basically to be there at this critical doorway.

Becoming Us

The true gauge of our education is not marketability, but who we have become.

- Jim Wallis

The 2020 commencement ceremonies around campuses around the world moved to virtual speeches in light of the COVID-19 pandemic. Surely those student's senior year was indelibly marked by distance learning, loss of personal contact, and traditional senior (high school) rituals. How will this shape who they become?

Our own lactation education has shaped us. Until recent changes in our credentialing process, we knew we would be expanding our knowledge base with CERPS, contact hours, and sitting for the IBLCE exam at least every 10 years. With each 5-year recertification, we became different people. Our life experience and our professional experience have shaped who we are today. Is there any old skin you'd like to shed? What do you celebrate about the person you've become?

Hopes home is at the innermost part of us.

- Reverend Doctor Cynthia Bourgeault

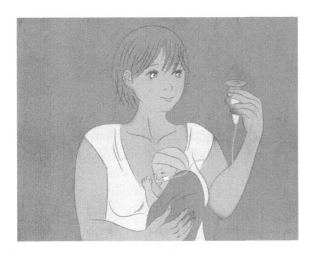

For some practitioners, lactation is a steppingstone to another career, sometimes related, sometimes altogether different. Whether you are in it for the long haul or this is a brief part of your career path, something resides at your deepest level that helps you discern your path. When you feel at a crossroads, when you feel enormously discouraged about the state of healthcare in your country or institution, when you're not sure you have it in you to continue, go to your inmost place of hope and listen. You'll know how to move forward.

In the same way, we invite mothers to listen to that place called hope and let it lead them on their lactation journey. In moments of doubt about continuing to pump or nurse, when they don't know if something is a phase or a permanent fixture, they will look for hope to be reflected in your eyes. That's so much better than advising because they will have found that where hope resides, their authentic self resides, and whatever they decide will bring peace.

Self-Care

Even purposeful giving must be replenished.

- Ann Morrow Lindbergh

My 7-year-old granddaughter explained how she stays fit; "Three things, Grandma: hard work, hard work, hard work." I could hardly contain my laughter. I think it bears repeating three times; it is hard work to take care of ourselves. It's so easy to put other's needs first and so easy to ignore our own. We'll get to it eventually.

Stop. Rest. Take care of yourself. Take care of yourself. Take care of yourself.

What is the meaning of life? To humbly and proudly return what you've been given.

- Unknown

What about your life's work has given you the most meaning for this one beautiful life you are living? Each bit of knowledge imparted, each act of promotion, support, and protection of breastfeeding hasn't left us with less. Yes, there are days, perhaps many days of fatigue, but we've wound up with more, haven't we? We are passing on our life work each day. I don't know if mentoring is in your job description, but I'm guessing that you do that formally and informally, both with parents and colleagues.

You are returning the gifts you've been given.

Well done, my friend, well done.

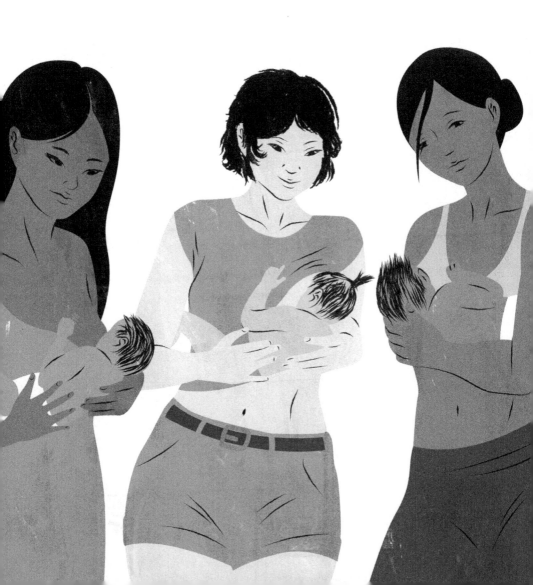

Under One Sky

Intimate Encounters with Moms and Babies by a Breastfeeding Consultant and Nurse

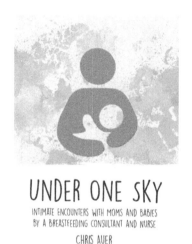

UNDER ONE SKY

INTIMATE ENCOUNTERS WITH MOMS AND BABIES
BY A BREASTFEEDING CONSULTANT AND NURSE

CHRIS AUER

Under One Sky recounts poignant encounters surrounding birth, breastfeeding, and the life circumstances of families from over 77 countries. As a lactation consultant, Chris Auer met with thousands of women as they began their mothering and breastfeeding journey, women from places as diverse as The Congo, Ecuador, Italy, and Nepal, as well as American women from all walks of life. The babies range from healthy, full-term to extremely premature. The mothers range from 12 to 52. Chris Auer has worked passionately to champion mothers on this segment of their life journey. In the retelling of their stories, we see the importance of meeting mothers where they are in the moment, with an accepting, listening presence. *Under One Sky* is beyond a memoir; it's a mosaic of their stories and reveals a poignant picture of our connectedness.

PraeclarusPress.com

Made in the USA
Monee, IL
18 May 2021